a guide to gonad discovery

22 WAYS TO HEAL HIM

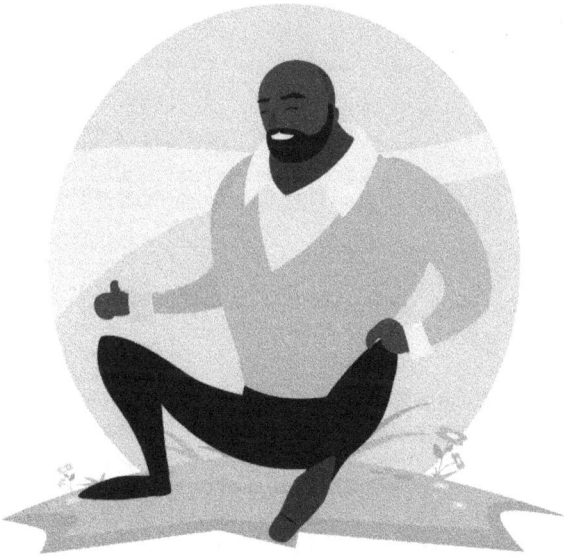

FELICIA GUY-LYNCH

Dedication

To all those striving to heal and maintain salvation

Preface

Yo! Where do I begin? Gender and sexuality are topics at an all-time high of sensitivity.

Still, there is a need more (now than ever) to heal the exchange between men and women.

With the help of some seasoned men currently in my inner circle, I am grateful for their honest insights. It is the foundation of this book.

When I wrote *22 Ways to Heal Her*, I desired to have one written for men as well.

Truth is, I am not a man. I am still trying to better establish healthy companionship with men to this day.

I've been writing since 2011 and I'm still learning.

Anywho, I hope you enjoy the complimentary sentiments of *22 Ways to Heal Him*.

Peace,

Felicia Guy-Lynch

Believe

What are your values? Where do they come from?

check within

Share Insight

Are you the pot calling the kettle black?

check your cypher

Forgive

Everyone is a villain in someone's story.
How can you heal the mind and body when you consciously
choose to nurse poison within your heart?

check out: theforgivenessproject.com

Abstain

You can't purge out if you keep letting the wrong energy in.
Is the right energy at the wrong time still the wrong energy?

check out: Man Heal Thyself: Journey to Optimal Wellness

Vent

The more you repress and suppress your emotions, the more you stress out your balls.

Process.

Write it out.

Talk it out.

Repeat.

call a friend. meet up somewhere

Prognosis

Don't get into the trap of self-diagnosis.
Follow up.
Get your prostate checked out man.

call your doctor to book an appointment

Counseling

Get trusted, professional help to unpack, make sense of, cope and overcome past trauma.

check out: therapyforblackmen.org

Recognize and Release Suppressed Emotions

Men cry too.

check out: menshealth.com

Herbs, Minerals & Other Supplements

check out: healthline.com/health/herbs-vitamins-supplements-testosterone-levels-balance

What are the benefits?

- Malaysian Ginseng
  - Increase libido
  - Enhance sports performance
  - Stimulate the production of androgen hormones, such as testosterone
- Ashwagandha
  - Increased sperm concentrations
  - Enhanced volume of ejaculate
  - Increased serum testosterone levels and improved sperm motility
- Vitamin D
  - Fight off bacteria and viruses
  - Absorb calcium into your bones
  - Increase testosterone levels
- Zinc
  - Produce DNA and genetic material
  - Repair the gastrointestinal tract
  - Boost testosterone levels for people with zinc deficiencies

Enema

What's is it and the benefits?

- An enema is a procedure that involves injecting a liquid or gas, into the rectum through the anus to either administer medication or flush out fecal matter
- It can help with treating ulcerative colitis, alleviating severe constipation and assisting medical professionals with giving a diagnosis

check out: badgut.org

Focus

Don't forget your blindspot too!

check your third eye

Exercise

check out: mensjournal.com/health-fitness/the-15-most-important-exercises-for-men

What are the benefits to each workout?

- <u>Banded Good Morning</u>: although this move looks like it would hurt your lower back, it in fact has the opposite effect. The good morning is a great developer for those muscles, and the use of a band makes it more like a physical therapy exercise than a traditional lift. Not only that, but this exercise will assist you in the squat, allowing you to load up more weight on the bar.

- <u>Back Squat</u>: Just like the deadlift, the barbell back squat hits just about every major muscle group there is in the body and is the king of leg-developing movements. Any athlete will tout the squat as the reason they run fast, jump high, and keep increasing in strength all over.

- <u>Medicine Ball Slam</u>: Some guys work for a lifetime to develop a ripped midsection like the fitness models we see in magazines. Others know the secret of disciplined eating and the best exercises for abs out there, none of which are a crunch or variation. The medicine ball slam carves out gorges in the midsection, making your abs look like a street map of midtown Manhattan and adds a good amount of cardio to your workout so you can maintain that look.

Assert Your Masculinity

Balance is key

Ionic
Foot Bath

What is it and the benefits?

- This process gives the hydrogen in the water a positive charge. The positive charge attracts the negatively charged toxins in your body. The ions in the foot bath water hold a charge that enables them to bind to heavy metals and toxins in your body. This allows the toxins to be pulled out through the bottoms of your feet

Color of the Water	Area of the Body Represented/Detoxified
Black	liver
Black Flecks	heavy metals
Blue	kidney
Brown	liver, tobacco, cellular debris
Green	gallbladder
Orange	joints
Red Flecks	cellular debris, blood clot material
Yellow	kidney, bladder, urinary tract, female/prostate area
Cheesy	candidas, fungal infections, most likely yeast
Foam	lymphatic drainage, mucus
Oil Floating	fat

check out: healthline.com

31

Lemon & Ginger

What are some benefits?
- Fights infection with its combined anti-inflammatory, anti-bacterial, anti-fungal, anti-diabetic, anti-cancer and anti-viral properties
- Reduces nausea
- Optimizes thyroid health

check out: emilykylenutrition.com

Check Your Flaws

Progression is way more important than pretending to be perfect

check the barometer of your self love

Bentonite Clay and Psyllium Husk

consult a health professional

What are some benefits?

The bentonite clay absorbs toxins and the psyllium husk scrubs out the corners of your intestines. This encourages the:

- Removal of plastics and heavy metals
- Reversal of radiation exposure
- Alleviation of symptoms associated with irritable bowel syndrome (IBS)

Colon Hydrotherapy

check out: yurielkaim.com

It is commonly referred to as a colonic irrigation or colon cleansing. It's similar to an enema but uses more liquid along with special herbs, enzymes or probiotics to accentuate the healing process.

Some of the benefits are that it stimulates bowel movement, increases your chances of fertility and helps to maintain a healthy pH level for your blood.

Fiber Intake

What are the different types?

Cellulose - insoluble fiber found in vegetables like cabbage that bind to other food particles to assist with bowel movement

Inulin - soluble fiber derived from chicory root found naturally in wheat like barley. It leaves you feeling fuller for longer by slowing down digestion

Pectin - soluble fiber found in vegetables like strawberries help reduce the glycemic response of foods by stalling glucose absorption. In other words, no sugar spikes

Beta-Glucans - a gel-forming type of soluble fiber found in foods like reishi mushrooms that easily gets broken down by the gut flora

Psyllium - a prebiotic, soluble fiber found in high-fiber cereals that help relieve constipation by softening bowels to help it pass

Lignin - an insoluble fiber that's part of the cell wall structure in plants such as avocados that may help to reduce the risk of developing colon cancer

Resistant Starch - a type of fiber found in legumes and beans that passes through the large intestine, protecting the GI tract from harmful bacteria

check out: cookinglight.com

Fermented Foods

What are the different types?

Lactic Acid Fermentation - relies on yeasts and bacteria to convert starches and sugars into lactic acid and contains live organisms (probiotics) E.g.) Sauerkraut, kombucha, kimchi and bread

Ethyl Alcohol Fermentation - uses yeast to break down starches and sugars to make wine and beer but does not contain live organisms

Acetic Acid Fermentation - vinegar is used to make fermented foods such as pickles

Overall, fermented foods protect the intestinal mucous membrane from leaking, alleviates symptoms in autoimmune disorders and plays a key role in helping your body maintain a healthy gut-brain relationship.

Testosterone Supplements

Keep estrogen levels at a low level

check out: healthline.com/nutrition/8-ways-to-boost-testosterone

Epsom Salt Bath

The two main ingredients of Epsom salt are magnesium and sulfate. The two combined stimulate detoxification.

Magnesium aids in the body's ability to remove toxins responsible for inflammation while also reducing swelling, stiffness and pain.

Sulfate makes releasing toxins easier.

Adding therapeutic oils such as lavender can make a detox bath more relaxing.

check out: medicalnewstoday.com